GASTROPARESIS DIET COOKBOOK FOR SENIORS

Nourishing Recipes and Lifestyle Tips for Gentle Digestion and Improved Well-Being; A Comprehensive Guide

Smart Desty

TABLE OF CONTENTS

INTRODUCTION

James, who was well into his seventies, had always been a lively and busy man. During his retirement, he played with his grandchildren, tended to his garden, and volunteered at the neighborhood animal shelter. However, during the previous 12 months, things had begun to shift. He started having stomach pain, bloating, and nausea all the time. His once voracious appetite diminished, and he started skipping meals out of fear of the agony they would cause.

James was given a gastroparesis diagnosis following multiple trips to the physician and a battery of testing. The announcement caused both relief and alarm. It felt overwhelming to think of having to manage a chronic ailment, but at least he had an explanation. His physician advised him to consult a dietician with expertise in gastroparesis and stressed the significance of making dietary adjustments to control his symptoms.

It was eye-opening for James to meet his nutritionist, Sarah, for the first time. She described how a unique diet was necessary to alleviate his discomfort due to his stomach's delayed emptying. They worked together to develop a diet plan that would be easy on his digestive system and give him the nutrients he need.

James, Sarah smiled comfortingly, the trick is to eat small, frequent meals and make low-fat, high-fiber food choices. This will facilitate faster food digestion in your stomach.

The modifications were difficult at first. James yearned for the crunchy salads he used to love and missed his huge meals of bacon and eggs. However, Sarah gave him more nourishing and easily digestible options. His new favorite breakfast was smoothies made with low-fat yogurt, soft fruits, and a little honey. He liked rich, calming blended vegetable soups instead of salads.

The largest change was figuring out how to make meals ahead of time. Sarah showed him how to prepare meals in bulk and freeze them so he would always have a gastroparesis-friendly meal available. This not only made things easier on a daily basis but also made it easier for him to maintain his new diet without feeling pressured.

Weeks later, James saw a noticeable improvement in his problems as the months went by. His bloating and nausea subsided, and he started to look forward to meals once more. Even the recipes from the Gastroparesis Diet Cookbook for Seniors that Sarah had suggested he try out.

One afternoon, Emily, James's granddaughter, came into the kitchen as she was making a pot of low-fat chicken and rice soup. What are you creating, grandpa? It has a wonderful aroma.

Emily, this soup is unique, James retorted while agitating the saucepan. It tastes great even though it's easy on my stomach. Do you want to assist me?

Emily excitedly accompanied him, and the two of them conversed and cooked. With wide eyes filled with excitement, Emily listened as James related stories about his early years. James was reminded of the significance of maintaining his health by such events. He desired to share in his family's life, be present for them, and make new memories.

Sarah called one day to see how James was doing. James, how are you feeling? Have you observed any modifications?

James remarked, I feel like a new man, with a tone of thankfulness. I had no idea how much my diet may affect my overall health. I'm enjoying my food again, not just eating to stay comfortable. And I have more energy now to do the things I enjoy.

Hearing this thrilled Sarah. That's fantastic, James! It all comes down to balance and paying attention to your body, remember? You've adjusted to these changes quite well.

James felt proud of himself as he thought back on his voyage. Changing to a gastroparesis diet had not only made his symptoms better, but it had also brought him back to enjoy cooking and eating. It made him appreciate life's little pleasures, such as eating with loved ones and feeling confident in his own flesh.

James went on to enjoy his new way of living with a fresh lease on life. He was more involved in voluntary work, gave his garden his all, and spent as much time as possible playing with his grandchildren. He felt as though his symptoms had been relieved, but the nutritional adjustments had given him a new lease on life.

Although James was aware that managing his gastroparesis will always be necessary, he was no longer intimidated by the idea. Equipped with an abundance of information, a reassuring nutritionist, and a cookbook brimming with delectable meals, he felt assured of his capacity to live a happy and meaningful life.

And so, knowing that he could control his condition and make the most of his golden years, James celebrated his modest wins with every meal he cooked and every day that went by.

It can be quite difficult to live with gastroparesis, particularly for seniors who also have other health issues. Every day might be difficult due to the discomfort, nausea, and dietary limitations, and it may seem impossible to locate delightful foods that are also appropriate for your condition. But you're not alone on this path, and you can make managing your gastroparesis through diet a manageable—even enjoyable—part of your everyday routine if you have the correct support.

This cookbook has been specifically created with seniors in mind, taking into account the special difficulties and dietary requirements associated with aging. Our bodies' nutritional needs change as we age, and our digestive systems may become more delicate. When these variables are combined with gastroparesis, it becomes imperative to plan ahead and make deliberate decisions in order to preserve health and wellbeing. This book aims to give you doable, tasty, and easily digestible recipes that will support you in managing your symptoms and make sure you get the nutrients you need.

Comprehend Gastropteriosis

One of the symptoms of gastroparesis is delayed stomach emptying. In order to transfer food into the small intestine for additional digestion, the stomach normally contracts. But in those who have gastroparesis, these contractions are either weak or nonexistent, which results in food staying in the stomach for longer than usual. Numerous symptoms, such as nausea, vomiting, bloating, and stomach discomfort, may result from this.

Although the precise etiology of gastroparesis is frequently unknown, it has been linked to diabetes, certain drugs, and other medical conditions. Because of the increased risk of malnutrition and the existence of other age-related health conditions, the condition can be especially problematic for seniors. It is essential to understand how to control gastroparesis with nutrition in order to enhance general health and quality of life.

Diet is Crucial for Managing Gastoresis

An important aspect of controlling gastroparesis is diet. The stomach's capacity to evacuate its contents is impaired, thus it's critical to eat foods high in nutrients and easy to digest. This entails emphasizing foods that are easier for the stomach to process, such as low-fat, low-fiber options. Additionally, it entails eating more frequently and in smaller portions to prevent overtaxing the digestive system.

It can be challenging for seniors to strike a balance between the dietary restrictions brought on by gastroparesis and the aging body's nutritional requirements. For seniors to keep their muscles, bones, and general vigor intact, they must consume enough protein, vitamins, and minerals. This cookbook is intended to assist you in overcoming these obstacles by providing recipes that are both appropriate for people with gastroparesis and specifically crafted to fulfill the dietary needs of senior citizens.

Using This Cookbook

This cookbook is broken up into multiple chapters, each of which focuses on a distinct facet of diet-based gastroparesis management. We start by going over the fundamentals of a diet for gastroparesis, including what foods to eat and avoid as well as advice on how to plan and prepare meals. You'll gain a strong basis for understanding how to choose foods that promote your health from this part.

You will find a number of recipes arranged by meal type (breakfast, lunch, supper, snacks, and desserts) after the introductory chapters. Every recipe is meant to be rich and filling, but also simple to make and easy on the digestive tract. A chapter on drinks is also included because it's crucial for people with gastroparesis to stay hydrated.

We've also included a chapter on particular diet considerations, which addresses frequent issues including controlling blood sugar in elderly diabetics and customizing recipes. This section will assist you in customizing your diet to meet your unique health needs.

The cookbook ends with lifestyle advice for managing gastroparesis, appendices with useful tools like meal planning templates and conversion charts, and a resources section with suggested reading and support groups. With a complete approach to managing your condition, these resources are meant to provide you with help that goes beyond just the recipes.

Regarding Seniors in Particular

You have certain dietary requirements as a senior, which should be considered when treating gastroparesis. You require more calcium, vitamin D, and protein as you age because of changes in your metabolism, muscle mass, and bone density. However, it may be challenging to get enough of these nutrients through diet and intestinal problems.

Taking these things into account, this cookbook provides meals that are high in nutrients and easy to digest, keeping you healthy. Nutrient-dense foods are important because they include more vitamins and minerals per calorie than other foods. Seniors, who might have decreased appetites but still need to achieve their nutritional demands, should pay special attention to this.

We also understand that a large number of seniors have fixed incomes and might not have easy access to fresh, premium ingredients. In light of this, we've included recipes that use inexpensive, easily accessible products as well as money-saving purchasing advice. Our intention is to simplify and keep the cost of a gastroparesis-friendly diet affordable for you.

Giving You the Ability to Take Charge of Your Health

Although having gastroparesis can often feel overwhelming, you can manage your health and enhance your quality of life if you have the correct information and resources. With its helpful tips and delectable recipes, this cookbook aims to empower you to manage gastroparesis more easily and joyfully.

Recall that each individual's experience with gastroparesis is unique, so what helps one person may not help another. It's critical to pay close attention to your body's needs and collaborate closely with your medical team to create a customized management plan for your illness. We hope that this cookbook will provide you the motivation and support you need to manage your gastroparesis successfully. It is simply one tool to aid you on your path.

We are honored that you have included our cookbook in your quest for better health. Along with tasty meals, we hope it gives you optimism and a sense of empowerment while you manage your gastroparesis. You are not by yourself, and by working together, we may somewhat ease the management of this situation.

Chapter 1: Understanding Gastroparesis

Your quality of life can be greatly impacted by having gastroparesis, particularly in regards to eating and digestion. It's essential to comprehend the fundamentals of a gastroparesis diet in order to control symptoms and preserve general health. You will find all the information you need in this chapter regarding gastroparesis, including symptoms and dietary recommendations to make your life easier.

Gastroparesis: What is it?

A persistent illness called gastroparesis impairs the stomach's capacity to release its contents slowly. A number of painful symptoms, such as nausea, vomiting, bloating, and stomach discomfort, can result from this delayed gastric emptying. Numerous variables, including diabetes, surgery, infections, and specific drugs, might contribute to the illness. Nevertheless, the precise cause is frequently still unknown.

The stomach muscles contract in a healthy digestive system to transfer food into the small intestine for additional processing and absorption. Due to weak or nonexistent contractions, food stays in the stomach longer than it should in patients with gastroparesis. As a result, solid lumps known as bezoars may form, further obstructing the digestive tract and aggravating symptoms.

Gastroparesis Symptoms

The degree of gastroparesis symptoms varies and can include:

- Sickness
- Regurgitating (usually from leftover food)
- Bloating
- Pain in the abdomen
- Early satiety (feeling satisfied soon)
- Appetite loss
- Weight loss
- Malnourishment

Your everyday life and general well-being may be greatly impacted by these symptoms. Gastroparesis is often managed with a mix of dietary modifications, medication, and occasionally surgery. Nonetheless, nutrition and symptom management are greatly influenced by diet.

Nutritional Guidelines for Gastroparesis Management

A gastroparesis-friendly diet entails modifying certain foods and eating habits. You can choose foods that are less likely to aggravate your symptoms and easier to digest by using the following tips.

1. Consume Light Meals Frequently

Eating smaller meals more frequently throughout the day is one of the most crucial dietary recommendations for treating gastroparesis. Try to have five or six modest meals per day rather than three large ones. This method assists in keeping your stomach from filling up too much, which can worsen symptoms and slow down digestion.

2. Select Foods Low in Fat

Low-fat foods are the best choice because fat slows down the emptying of the stomach. Steer clear of full-fat dairy products, high-fat meats, and fried foods. Select lean proteins, dairy products that are low in fat or fat free, and cooking techniques like baking, grilling, or steaming instead.

Low-fat meal options include, for example:
- A chicken breast without skin
- Turkey
- Trimmed beef or pork portions
- Fat or low-fat-free yogurt
- Low-fat or skim milk
- Low-fat cheese

3. Select Foods Low in Fiber

Although high-fiber diets might be difficult to digest and exacerbate symptoms of gastroparesis, fiber is generally good for digestion. Select foods low in fiber, such as white rice, bread, and well-cooked veggies devoid of seeds or skins.

Low-fiber food options include, for example:
- White bread - White rice
- Simple pasta
- Skinless, well-cooked veggies (such as green beans and carrots)
- Peel-free canned fruits (peaches, pears, etc.)

4. Give Food a Good Chew

Enough chewing of food prior to swallowing can facilitate easier digestion. Your stomach can handle smaller food particles more easily, which lessens the chance of discomfort and increases the effectiveness of gastric emptying.

5. Steer clear of foods high in fiber and gas.

Bloating and discomfort can be brought on by some gassy and high-fiber diets. Steer clear of items such as beans, cabbage, broccoli, and other cruciferous vegetables. Whole grains, raw veggies, and legumes can also be problematic. Rather, concentrate on items that are simple to digest and won't make your symptoms worse.

6. Maintain Hydration

Although it's important to stay hydrated, consuming a lot of liquid at once may cause your stomach to fill up too soon. Drink liquids all during the day as opposed to all at once. Clear broths and soups, as well as non-carbonated beverages, are ideal choices. Steer clear of fizzy drinks since they can produce gas and bloating.

7. Take into Account Pureed or Liquid Foods

It may be required to consume pureed or liquid foods in severe cases of gastroparesis. These foods can guarantee that you get enough nutrition and are easier to digest. Meal replacement shakes, pureed soups, and smoothies can all be helpful. Speak with a nutritionist or your healthcare professional to determine what solutions will best suit your nutritional needs.

8. Include Foods High in Calories but Low in Volume

Selecting foods that offer a high calorie and nutrient content in a short amount of food is crucial because gastroparesis can cause weight loss and malnutrition. By doing this, you may keep your weight and nutritional condition stable without putting too much food in your stomach.

Foods high in calories but low in volume include: - Nut butters, when consumed in moderation
- Hummus - Avocado - Low-fat cheese
- Smoothies high in nutrients

9. Keep an eye on your blood sugar levels

Controlling blood sugar levels is essential for diabetics, particularly since gastroparesis can result in erratic blood sugar fluctuations. In close collaboration with your healthcare professional, keep an eye on and regulate your blood sugar levels. Make necessary adjustments to your diet and medication regimen.

10. Document Your Diet

Maintaining a meal journal can assist you in determining the foods that cause your symptoms. Keep a journal of your food intake, meal timings, and any symptoms you encounter. You might start to see trends over time that will guide your eating decisions.

Foods to Incorporate and Exclude

It is crucial to know which foods to include and avoid in your diet in order to effectively manage your gastroparesis. Here's a closer look at a few particular foods and how they affect your digestive system.

Foods You Should Eat

- Lean Proteins: Tofu, fish, eggs (especially egg whites), skinless chicken, lean beef, and pork tenderloin.
Low-fat dairy products include skim milk, fat-free or low-fat yogurt, and low-fat cheese.
Low-fiber cereals, white bread, white rice, and plain pasta are examples of refined grains.
- Well-Cooked Vegetables: Skinless potatoes, carrots, zucchini, and green beans.
- Soft or Canned Fruits: Bananas, applesauce, pears, peaches.
- Smoothies and Shakes: Concocted of fruit, protein powder, and low-fat yogurt.

- Pure Soups and Broths: Miso soup, vegetable broth, and chicken broth.

Avoided Foods

High-Fat Foods: Fried foods, meats with high fat content, dairy products with whole milk, and creamy sauces.

- High-Fiber Foods: Nuts, seeds, raw veggies, legumes, and whole grains.

Brussels sprouts, cauliflower, broccoli, and cabbage are examples of gassy vegetables.

Seeds and Nuts: Can cause bezoars and be difficult to digest.

- Carbonated Drinks: Beer, soda, and sparkling water.

- Tough Meats: Meats that are hard to chew and digest, such as steak and pork chops.

Advice on Organizing and Preparing Meals

Organizing and preparing meals is essential to managing gastroparesis. Here are some pointers to get you going:

1. Make a plan beforehand

Spend some time organizing your weekly meal plan. By doing this, you can make sure you have all the components you need on hand and prevent impulsive judgments that could result in bad nutritional choices.

2. Prepare Meals in Bulk and Freeze Them

Make bigger quantities of gastroparesis-friendly food and parcel it out for freezing. This eliminates the hassle of daily cooking and makes it simpler to have a healthy meal available when you need it.

3. Make Preparation Easy with Kitchen Tools
Invest in kitchen appliances that will make meal preparation easier, such a food processor for pureeing veggies, a blender for smoothies, and a slow cooker for soups and stews.

4. Pay Attention to Portion Sizes
Reduce the size of your dishes and bowls to aid in portion control. Eating more often and in smaller portions will help keep your stomach from getting too full and slowing down digestion.

5. Maintain Order
Maintain a well-stocked and orderly kitchen that is suitable for people with gastroparesis. This lessens the urge to eat foods that could cause symptoms and makes it simpler to follow your diet.

Consulting a Dietician
In order to effectively manage gastroparesis, a licensed dietitian can be a great resource. They can assist you in developing a customized meal plan that takes into account your dietary preferences and symptoms in addition to satisfying your nutritional demands. Frequent check-ins with a dietician can also offer continuing assistance and diet modifications as required.

A gastroparesis diet is easy to understand, and knowing this will help you manage your illness and live a better quality of life. You may take charge of your symptoms and preserve your general health by adhering to these dietary recommendations, selecting the appropriate foods, and collaborating closely with your medical team. We'll go over detailed meal plans, recipes, and advice in the upcoming chapters to help you incorporate these ideas into your everyday life. Recall that each person's experience with gastroparesis is distinct, so it's critical to pay attention to your body's signals and modify as necessary.

Chapter 2: Senior's Nutrition

Nutritional demands vary with age. It might be especially difficult for seniors with gastroparesis to balance these needs with the dietary restrictions imposed by their disease. This chapter examines the particular dietary needs of elderly people, how to maintain a balanced diet, and the significance of vitamins and supplements for general health and wellbeing.

Seniors' Nutritional Needs

Numerous physiological changes brought on by aging impact the needs for nutrition. Reduced muscular mass, a changed metabolism, a diminished ability to absorb nutrients, and adjustments to hunger are some of these alterations. The problem is compounded for elderly patients with gastroparesis because the illness might result in additional nutritional deficits because of reduced food intake and impaired digestion.

1. Needs for Protein

For muscular mass to be maintained—which normally declines with age—protein is essential. Sustaining mobility and independence requires maintaining muscle strength and function, which is aided by an adequate protein consumption. High-quality protein sources, such as lean meats, fish, eggs, dairy products, lentils, and tofu, should be a goal for seniors' diets. On the other hand, it's crucial to stay away from high-fat meats and select readily digestible protein sources for those with gastroparesis.

2. Vitamin D and Calcium

For healthy bones, calcium and vitamin D are essential. People's capacity to absorb calcium declines with age, and the skin's capacity to produce vitamin D from sunshine is diminished. This may result in weaker bones and a higher chance of fractures. Good sources of calcium include dairy products, fish such as salmon and sardines, leafy green vegetables, and fortified plant milks. Supplements, cautious sun exposure, and fortified foods are good sources of vitamin D.

3. Texture

Although high-fiber diets might be challenging for people with gastroparesis to digest, fiber is essential for digestive health. Striking a balance between preventing constipation and easing the symptoms of gastroparesis is crucial. Fruits in cans, refined grains, and thoroughly cooked veggies without skins are examples of low-fiber foods. Supplements containing soluble fiber, such as psyllium, may also be advantageous and simpler to handle.

4. Drinking Plenty of Water
Seniors are more likely to become dehydrated because they may have a loss in renal function and a diminished sense of thirst. Digestion and general health are dependent on

adequate hydration. Large amounts of liquid, however, might make the symptoms of gastroparesis worse. Drinking small amounts of fluids throughout the day as opposed to a high one-time intake will help you stay hydrated without feeling queasy. Water, herbal teas, clear soups, and broths are all healthy choices.

5. Minerals and Vitamins

The use and absorption of some vitamins and minerals can be impacted by aging. Given the importance of vitamins B12, B6, and folate for nerve health and red blood cell synthesis, seniors may require larger doses of these nutrients. Although they might be absorbed less effectively, iron, magnesium, and zinc are all vital. To help achieve these nutritional needs, a diversified diet full of fruits, vegetables, whole grains, lean meats, and fortified foods is recommended. To guarantee enough consumption, people with gastroparesis might need to take supplements.

Maintaining a Balanced Diet while Balancing Nutrients

Careful planning and inventiveness are needed to strike a balance between the limitations imposed by gastroparesis and the requirement for a sufficient diet. The idea is to serve nutrient-dense, easily digestible foods that don't make symptoms worse.

1. Light Dinners Often

Increasing the frequency of smaller meals throughout the day can help control the symptoms of gastroparesis and guarantee a consistent nutrient intake. By taking this method, the stomach is kept from filling up too much, which might impede gastric emptying and result in discomfort.

2. Foods High in Nutrients

Select foods that are minimal in volume yet abundant in vital nutrients. This tactic aids in achieving dietary requirements without packing the stomach. Smoothies made with fruits, low-fat yogurt, and a scoop of protein powder are a few examples.
- Soups made from pureed vegetables, lean meats, and lentils.
- Soft-cooked grains, such as quinoa or oats.

3. Steer clear of foods high in fat and fiber

Foods heavy in fat and fiber can impede stomach emptying and exacerbate the symptoms of gastroparesis. Choose low-fat cooking techniques including poaching, baking, grilling, or steaming. Make sure to choose low-fiber foods such as boiled veggies and refined grains.

4. Include Pureed and Liquid Foods

Foods that are liquid or pureed can be rich in nutrients and are typically easy to digest. Include foods in your diet such as smoothies, blended soups, pureed fruits and vegetables, and meal replacement shakes. These can give vital nutrients without making you uncomfortable.

5. Observe and Modify

To monitor your diet and how it impacts your symptoms, keep a food journal. Finding trigger foods and patterns might be aided by this. Based on your research, modify your diet; for individualized advice, speak with a nutritionist.

Vitamins and Supplements

It can be difficult for elderly people with gastroparesis to obtain all the nutrients they need from food alone. It could be necessary to take vitamins and supplements to promote general health and repair nutritional gaps.

1. Supplemental vitamins

Ensuring proper consumption of vital vitamins and minerals can be facilitated by taking a senior-specific daily multivitamin. Because older persons frequently require higher levels of vitamin B12, vitamin D, and calcium, look for formulations that incorporate these nutrients.

2. Supplements with Protein

Without requiring a lot of food, protein supplements like whey protein powder or protein shakes can assist satisfy protein needs. These supplements can be added to drinks, soups, and smoothies. They come in a variety of flavors.

3. Supplementing with Calcium and Vitamin D

Supplements of calcium and vitamin D may be required to support bone health. Due to its easier absorption, elderly are frequently advised to take calcium citrate. Supplementing with vitamin D3 can help guarantee sufficient levels of vitamin D, particularly for people who get little sun exposure.

4. Supplements with Fiber

Without the bulk of high-fiber foods, soluble fiber supplements like psyllium husk can assist preserve digestive health. To assist avoid constipation, these supplements can be added to diet or combined with water.

5. Fatty Acids Omega-3

Omega-3 fatty acids can promote heart and brain function and have anti-inflammatory qualities. Seniors may benefit from taking fish oil supplements or omega-3 plant-based supplements like flaxseed oil.

6. Supplemental Liver

Probiotics can enhance digestive health by supporting a balanced gut microbiota. A balanced gut flora can be maintained with the aid of probiotic pills or meals like yogurt, kefir, and fermented vegetables.

7. B vitamins and iron

Red blood cell formation and energy levels depend on iron and B vitamins. To avoid shortages, seniors—especially those who eat little meat—may require iron and B vitamin supplements.

Consulting a Dietician

When it comes to controlling gastroparesis and making sure you're getting enough nutrition, a qualified dietitian can be a great help. They can evaluate your nutritional status, help design balanced meal plans, and offer tailored dietary suggestions.

1. Tailored Food Schedules

A nutritionist can create meal plans that are customized to your tastes and requirements. They can assist you in avoiding trigger foods, controlling portion sizes, and incorporating foods high in nutrients.

2. Continuous Assistance and Observation

Consultations with a nutritionist on a regular basis can help you monitor your progress, alter your diet as needed, and handle any issues. They can also support you in overcoming obstacles and maintaining motivation.

3. Learning and Materials

Dietitians are excellent resources for information on managing gastroparesis and nutrition. They can provide you with tools to help you achieve your nutritional objectives, like meal ideas, cooking advice, and supplement information.

It is difficult but possible to strike a balance between the dietary constraints of gastroparesis and the nutritional requirements of aging. You may preserve your health and well-being by being aware of the special needs of seniors, including nutrient-dense foods in your diet, and taking vitamins and supplements as needed. Engaging with a dietitian can offer tailored direction and assistance, guaranteeing that your dietary requirements are fulfilled while controlling the symptoms of gastroparesis. We will go over particular meal plans, recipes, and useful hints in the upcoming chapters to help you incorporate these ideas into your everyday life and have a more satisfying and nutrient-dense diet.

Chapter 3: Making and Preparing Meals

Meal preparation and planning are essential for senior citizens with gastroparesis to manage symptoms and preserve nutritional health. This chapter explores the methods and useful advice to assist you in creating and cooking meals that are tasty, well-balanced, and easy to digest. We'll go through the fundamentals of meal planning, batch cooking, conscientious grocery shopping, and the value of kitchen appliances in streamlining the cooking process.

The Value of Meal Preparation

Planning your meals well ensures that you have the right foods on hand and lessens the anxiety associated with making meal choices, which helps you manage gastroparesis. It also aids in avoiding impulsive meal decisions that could not suit your nutritional requirements.

1. Organized Consumption

Small, regular meals on an organized eating plan can help control symptoms and keep the stomach from getting overly full. Instead of three major meals, plan for five to six smaller meals or snacks throughout the day. Better digestion and nutrition absorption are supported by this strategy.

2. Nutritious Diet

Efficient meal preparation guarantees that your diet is well-rounded and contains all the essential components. To make sure you obtain the proper balance of proteins, carbs, fats, vitamins, and minerals, concentrate on combining a variety of foods from different groups.

3. Cut Down on Food Wastage

Meal preparation in advance minimizes food waste. Knowing what you're going to eat and when can help you to minimize waste and spoilage by allowing you to buy only the ingredients you need and use them effectively.

Essentials of Meal Planning

Understanding your dietary requirements, selecting suitable recipes, and planning your meals and snacks are all part of creating a meal plan. The following are crucial actions for meal planning to be successful for elderly patients with gastroparesis:

1. Determine What You Need to Eat

Start by determining your nutritional needs and any dietary restrictions that may be unique to your case of gastroparesis. Take into account how many calories you require, how much protein you eat, and any vitamins or minerals you may be lacking. A customized evaluation can be obtained by speaking with a dietician.

2. Select Fitting Recipes

Choose recipes that support the management of your gastroparesis and your nutritional requirements. Seek for foods that are easy to digest, low in fat and fiber. Smoothies, soups that have been pureed, and soft, well-cooked dishes are great choices.

3. Make Weekly Meal Plans

Make a weekly menu with all of your meals and snacks on it. Put the schedule for each day—breakfast, lunch, dinner, and snacks—in writing. Make sure the items in your menu are diverse in order to avoid boredom and encourage a well-rounded diet.

4. Create an Inventory

After you've decided on your menu, make a thorough shopping list. Make sure you have enough ingredients for each meal and snack during the week by including all the ingredients you'll need. Follow your list to prevent buying extraneous products.

5. Get Ready in Advance

Make dishes or ingredients in advance if possible. Prepare veggies in advance, cook proteins in large quantities, and divide snacks. You can save time and maintain your food plan more easily by doing this preparation.

Cooking in Bulk and Freezing

Meal prep in bulk and freezing can save the lives of elderly patients suffering from gastroparesis. This method keeps gastroparesis-friendly meals readily available, which minimizes the amount of cooking you have to do each day and makes it easier for you to follow your diet.

The advantages of batch cooking

There are many advantages to batch cooking:
 Convenience: Less time and effort are required to prepare meals every day.
Consistency: Make sure you always provide meals that are suitable for people with gastroparesis.
- Cost-Effective: Cooking big batches of food and purchasing ingredients in bulk can save money.

2. Organizing Your Cooking in Bulk

To begin batch cooking, take the following actions:
- Select Recipes: Pick a couple of your favorite recipes that work well for large quantities of cooking. Purees, casseroles, stews, and soups are all excellent choices.
- Plan Portions: Determine how much food to serve by consulting your meal plan. For the most part, small, individual amounts work best while controlling gastroparesis.
Time of Schedule: Allocate a particular day or time every week to cooking in bulk. Make sure you have adequate time for meal preparation, cooling, and packaging.

3. Meal Preservation and Freezing

To keep your meals safe and of high quality, you must freeze and store them properly:
- Use Airtight Containers: To avoid freezer burn and contamination, store meals in airtight containers.
Label and Date: Write the name of the meal and the preparation date on the label of each container. This guarantees that you eat the older meals first and keeps you aware of what you have.
Freeze Correctly: Let food cool fully before freezing. To preserve quality, keep them in the freezer's coldest section.

4. Tips for Reheating

To guarantee safety and maintain flavor when reheating frozen meals, adhere to these guidelines:

- Safely Thaw: Use your microwave's defrost function or refrigerate meals to thaw them. Don't let food thaw at room temperature.

Reheat Evenly: To guarantee even heating, stir the food halfway through the warming process. Make sure the internal temperature reaches 165°F (74°C) by using a food thermometer.

Incorporate Wetness: Food can become dry when reheated, particularly pureed meals. To keep things moist, add a little water, broth, or sauce.

Conscientious Food Buying

Choosing the appropriate items, paying attention to labels, and budgeting are all part of smart grocery shopping. Here are some pointers to help you have more productive and successful shopping trips:

1. Use a list when shopping

Shop with a detailed list that is based on your food plan at all times. This aids in maintaining concentration and preventing impulsive purchases that might not be in line with your nutritional requirements.

2. Examine the Labels

It's crucial to read food labels if you have gastroparesis. Select low-fat and low-fiber goods; steer clear of those that contain artificial substances or added sweeteners. Make sure the serving sizes and nutritional facts meet your dietary needs by checking them.

3. Select Both Frozen and Fresh Produce

While fresh is best, frozen fruits and veggies are also great choices. To preserve the majority of their nutrients, they are frequently plucked and frozen at their ripest. Additionally, frozen choices may be more affordable and have a longer shelf life.

4. Steer clear of processed foods.

The symptoms of gastroparesis might be made worse by the high fat, fiber, and artificial ingredient content of processed meals. Whenever possible, choose whole, minimally processed foods.

5. Perimeter Shopping

Fresh vegetables, dairy products, meats, and seafood are usually found along the perimeter of the grocery store. Compared to the inner aisles, which are frequently stocked with processed and packaged goods, these sections provide a greater selection of whole foods.

6. Cost-Effective Advice

It's not always expensive to eat healthily. Here are some pointers for controlling your shopping spending:
- Buy in Bulk: Stock up on basics like pasta, rice, and canned foods.
- Make Use of Coupons and Sales: Reduce the cost of groceries by using coupons, discounts, and sales.
- Organize Seasonal Dinners: Select seasonal produce because it is frequently less expensive and more readily available.

Crucial Utensils for the Kitchen

Meal preparation may be more fun and easier with the correct kitchen utensils. You may cook meals that are suitable for someone with gastroparesis by using the following key tools:

1. Mixing apparatus

A good blender is essential for creating soups, purees, and smoothies. Seek for a blender with strong blades that can blend a wide range of substances together smoothly and without lumps.

2. Food Preparation Equipment

When chopping, slicing, and pureeing food, a food processor can save time and labor. It comes in particularly handy when preparing big batches of veggies, grinding nuts and seeds, or kneading dough.

3. Delicate Cooker

For preparing soups, stews, and casseroles that need to cook for extended periods of time, a slow cooker is ideal. You may set it and forget about it, giving you more time for other pursuits.

4. Basket for Steamer

Vegetables can be cooked with a steamer basket and still retain their nutrients. Vegetables that are steamed maintain their flavor and texture while being easier to digest.

5. Measurement Spoons and Cups

To manage portion amounts and follow recipes, accuracy in measurement is essential. Purchase a high-quality set of measuring spoons and cups to guarantee uniformity in your cooking.

6. Containers for Storage

For meal preparation and batch cooking, it is imperative to have an assortment of storage containers. Select containers that are freezer-friendly, safe to use in the microwave, and simple to label.

Useful Cooking Advice

Here are some more helpful culinary hints to assist you in preparing meals that are suitable for gastroparesis:

1. Employ Low-Fat Cooking Techniques

Choose for culinary techniques like baking, grilling, steaming, or poaching that call for little to no additional fat. These techniques aid in maintaining low fat diets, which is essential for the management of gastroparesis.

2. Include Spices and Herbs

Instead of depending solely on high-fat sauces or condiments, use herbs and spices to enhance the flavor of your food. Dried spices, citrus zest, and fresh herbs can give your food more nuance and richness.

3. Prepare Vegetables in--Detail

Raw or undercooked veggies are more difficult to digest than cooked ones. Vegetables that are steamed, boiled, or baked until tender can help ease gastrointestinal distress.

4. Try Different Textures

Some textures may be difficult for someone with gastroparesis to tolerate. Try out various textures to see one suits you the best. Foods can be made easier to consume and digest by pureeing, mashing, or finely cutting them.

5. Steer clear of excess

Reducing the size of your meals can help avoid the symptoms of gastroparesis. Dinners should be served on smaller plates to prevent going back for seconds. It's critical to pay attention to your body's signals of hunger and fullness.

To manage gastroparesis and make sure you obtain the nutrients you need to stay healthy, meal planning and preparation are essential. You can make cooking and eating more pleasurable and doable by employing necessary kitchen gear, meal planning, batch cooking, and smart shopping.

Chapter 4: Healthy Breakfast Recipes

Below are 15 Breakfast Recipes for a Gastroparesis Diet for Seniors

1. Creamy Oatmeal with Bananas

Ingredients:
- 1 cup quick oats
- 2 cups water
- 1/2 cup milk or milk alternative
- 1 ripe banana, mashed
- 1 tsp honey (optional)
- Pinch of cinnamon

Instructions:
1. Bring water to a boil in a pot.
2. Add oats and reduce heat to simmer.
3. Cook for 5 minutes, stirring occasionally.
4. Stir in milk and mashed banana.
5. Cook for another 2-3 minutes until creamy.
6. Add honey and cinnamon if desired.
7. Serve warm.
- Prep Time: 5 minutes
- Cook Time: 10 minutes
- **Nutritional Composition (per serving):**
  - Calories: 220
  - Protein: 7g
  - Fat: 3g
  - Carbohydrates: 44g
  - Fiber: 4g

2. Smoothie Bowl with Greek Yogurt

Ingredients:
- 1/2 cup Greek yogurt
- 1/2 cup almond milk
- 1/2 cup frozen berries
- 1/2 ripe banana
- 1 tbsp honey
- 1 tbsp chia seeds (optional)

Instructions:
1. Blend Greek yogurt, almond milk, frozen berries, banana, and honey until smooth.
2. Pour into a bowl and sprinkle with chia seeds if using.

- Prep Time: 5 minutes
- Cook Time: None
- Nutritional Composition (per serving):
  - Calories: 250
  - Protein: 12g
  - Fat: 5g
  - Carbohydrates: 38g
  - Fiber: 5g

3. Scrambled Eggs with Spinach

Ingredients:
- 2 eggs
- 1/4 cup milk or milk alternative
- 1/4 cup baby spinach, chopped
- Salt and pepper to taste
- 1 tsp olive oil

Instructions:
1. Whisk eggs and milk in a bowl.
2. Heat olive oil in a pan over medium heat.
3. Add spinach and cook until wilted.
4. Pour in the egg mixture and cook, stirring constantly, until scrambled.
5. Season with salt and pepper.

- Prep Time: 5 minutes
- Cook Time: 5 minutes
- Nutritional Composition (per serving):
  - Calories: 180
  - Protein: 12g
  - Fat: 13g
  - Carbohydrates: 3g
  - Fiber: 1g

4. Apple Cinnamon Smoothie

Ingredients:
- 1 apple, peeled and cored
- 1/2 cup Greek yogurt
- 1/2 cup almond milk
- 1 tsp cinnamon
- 1 tbsp honey

Instructions:
1. Blend apple, Greek yogurt, almond milk, cinnamon, and honey until smooth.

- Prep Time: 5 minutes   - Cook Time: None
- Nutritional Composition (per serving):
  - Calories: 200   - Protein: 10g
  - Fat: 3g   - Carbohydrates: 36g   - Fiber: 4g

5. Banana Rice Pudding

Ingredients:
- 1/2 cup cooked rice
- 1/2 cup milk or milk alternative
- 1 ripe banana, mashed
- 1 tsp vanilla extract
- 1 tbsp honey

Instructions:
1. Combine cooked rice and milk in a saucepan.
2. Cook over medium heat until thickened.
3. Stir in mashed banana, vanilla extract, and honey.

4. Serve warm or chilled.

- Prep Time: 5 minutes - Cook Time: 10 minutes
- Nutritional Composition (per serving):
  - Calories: 230   - Protein: 5g
  - Fat: 3g   - Carbohydrates: 47g
  - Fiber: 2g

6. Avocado Toast with Egg

Ingredients:
  - 1 slice whole grain bread
  - 1/2 ripe avocado
  - 1 boiled egg, sliced
  - Salt and pepper to taste

Instructions:
  1. Toast the bread.
  2. Mash the avocado and spread it on the toast.
  3. Top with sliced boiled egg.
  4. Season with salt and pepper.

- Prep Time: 5 minutes   - Cook Time: 5 minutes
- Nutritional Composition (per serving):
  - Calories: 250
  - Protein: 10g
  - Fat: 18g
  - Carbohydrates: 20g
  - Fiber: 7g

7. Blueberry Chia Pudding

Ingredients:
- 1/4 cup chia seeds
- 1 cup almond milk
- 1/2 cup blueberries
- 1 tbsp honey

Instructions:
1. Combine chia seeds and almond milk in a bowl.
2. Stir in blueberries and honey.
3. Refrigerate overnight or for at least 4 hours.

- Prep Time: 5 minutes
- Cook Time: None (refrigeration time required)
- Nutritional Composition (per serving):
  - Calories: 220   - Protein: 6g   - Fat: 9g
  - Carbohydrates: 32g   - Fiber: 10g

8. Cottage Cheese with Peaches

Ingredients:
- 1 cup low-fat cottage cheese
- 1/2 cup canned peaches in juice, drained and chopped
- 1 tbsp honey

Instructions:
1. Combine cottage cheese, chopped peaches, and honey in a bowl.
2. Mix well and serve.

- Prep Time: 5 minutes   - Cook Time: None
- Nutritional Composition (per serving):
  - Calories: 180   - Protein: 15g   - Fat: 2g
  - Carbohydrates: 28g   - Fiber: 1g

9. Soft-Boiled Eggs with Toast Soldiers

Ingredients:
- 2 eggs
- 2 slices whole grain bread
- Salt and pepper to taste

Instructions:
1. Bring a pot of water to a boil.
2. Gently lower the eggs into the water and boil for 6 minutes.
3. Remove eggs and place in cold water for 1 minute.
4. Toast the bread and cut into strips.
5. Serve eggs with toast soldiers for dipping.

- Prep Time: 5 minutes
- Cook Time: 6 minutes
- Nutritional Composition (per serving):
  - Calories: 240
  - Protein: 15g
  - Fat: 11g
  - Carbohydrates: 20g
  - Fiber: 3g

10. Rice Cakes with Almond Butter and Banana

Ingredients:
- 2 rice cakes
- 2 tbsp almond butter
- 1 banana, sliced

Instructions:
1. Spread almond butter on rice cakes.
2. Top with banana slices.

- Prep Time: 5 minutes - Cook Time: None
- Nutritional Composition (per serving):
  - Calories: 250
  - Protein: 6g
  - Fat: 12g
  - Carbohydrates: 32g
  - Fiber: 4g

11. Yogurt Parfait with Honey

Ingredients:
- 1 cup Greek yogurt
- 1/2 cup granola
- 1 tbsp honey

Instructions:
1. Layer Greek yogurt and granola in a glass.
2. Drizzle with honey.

- Prep Time: 5 minutes   - Cook Time: None
- Nutritional Composition (per serving):
  - Calories: 300   - Protein: 15g   - Fat: 10g
  - Carbohydrates: 38g   - Fiber: 4g

12. Pumpkin Smoothie

Ingredients:
- 1/2 cup canned pumpkin
- 1/2 cup Greek yogurt
- 1/2 cup almond milk
- 1 tsp pumpkin pie spice
- 1 tbsp honey

Instructions:
1. Blend canned pumpkin, Greek yogurt, almond milk, pumpkin pie spice, and honey until smooth.

- Prep Time: 5 minutes   - Cook Time: None
- Nutritional Composition (per serving):
  - Calories: 180
  - Protein: 10g
  - Fat: 3g
  - Carbohydrates: 30g
  - Fiber: 4g

13. Pear and Cottage Cheese

Ingredients:
- 1 cup low-fat cottage cheese
- 1 pear, peeled and chopped
- 1 tbsp honey

Instructions:
1. Combine cottage cheese, chopped pear, and honey in a bowl.

2. Mix well and serve.

- Prep Time: 5 minutes   - Cook Time: None
- Nutritional Composition (per serving):
  - Calories: 190
  - Protein: 15g
  - Fat: 2g
  - Carbohydrates: 30g
  - Fiber: 4g

14. Rice Porridge with Berries

Ingredients:
  - 1/2 cup cooked rice
  - 1/2 cup milk or milk alternative
  - 1/2 cup mixed berries
  - 1 tbsp honey

Instructions:
  1. Combine cooked rice and milk in a saucepan.
  2. Cook over medium heat until thickened.
  3. Stir in mixed berries and honey.
  4. Serve warm.

- Prep Time: 5 minutes   - Cook Time: 10 minutes
- Nutritional Composition (per serving):
  - Calories: 230
  - Protein: 6g
  - Fat: 3g
  - Carbohydrates: 45g
  - Fiber: 3g

15. Spinach and Feta Omelette

Ingredients:
- 2 eggs
- 1/4 cup milk or milk alternative
- 1/4 cup baby spinach, chopped
- 2 tbsp feta cheese, crumbled
- Salt and pepper to taste
- 1 tsp olive oil

Instructions:
1. Whisk eggs and milk in a bowl.
2. Heat olive oil in a pan over medium heat.
3. Add spinach and cook until wilted.
4. Pour in the egg mixture and cook until set.
5. Sprinkle with feta cheese and fold the omelette.
6. Season with salt and pepper.

- Prep Time: 5 minutes
- Cook Time: 5 minutes
- Nutritional Composition (per serving):
  - Calories: 220
  - Protein: 14g
  - Fat: 16g
  - Carbohydrates: 3g
  - Fiber: 1g

Chapter 5: Lunch Recipes

15 Lunch Recipes for Gastroparesis Diet

1. Soup with Chicken and Rice

Ingredients:
- 1 diced carrot;
- 1 celery stalk;
- 1/2 cup cooked white rice;
- 1/2 cup cooked shredded chicken;
- 2 cups low-sodium chicken broth;
- Salt and pepper to taste;
- 1 tsp olive oil

Directions:
1. In a pot over medium heat, warm the olive oil.
2. Add the celery and carrot and sauté until tender.
3. Include the chicken broth and heat through.
4. Include rice and cooked chicken.
5. Let it simmer for ten minutes.
6. Add pepper and salt for seasoning.

Cook Time: 20 minutes - Prep Time: 10 minutes
- Nutritional Composition (per serving): - 250 calories
  - 18g of protein
  - 4g of fat
  - 35g of carbohydrates
  - 2g of fiber

2. Rich Tomato Soup

Ingredients:

- One 14.5-ounce can of diced tomatoes;
- one cup of low-sodium chicken broth;
- half a cup of heavy cream
- One teaspoon of sugar
- To taste, add salt and pepper
- 1 tablespoon of olive oil

Directions:

1. In a pot over medium heat, warm the olive oil.
2. Include the chicken broth and diced tomatoes.
3. Let it simmer for ten minutes.
4. Use a blender to puree the soup until it's smooth.
5. Stir in sugar and heavy cream.
6. Add pepper and salt for seasoning.

Cook Time: 15 minutes - Prep Time: 5 minutes
- Nutritional Composition (per serving):
  - 200 calories
  - 4g of protein
  - 15g of fat
  - 15g of carbohydrates
  - 3g of fiber

3. Tuna Salad Wrap

Ingredients:
- One can (5 ounces) of drained tuna in water
– 2 tablespoons mayonnaise
- One tablespoon of Greek yogurt
- One teaspoon of lemon juice
One tablespoon of finely chopped celery
- One whole wheat tortilla - Salt and pepper to taste

Directions:
1. In a bowl, combine tuna, Greek yogurt, mayonnaise, lemon juice, and celery.
2. Add pepper and salt for seasoning.
3. Cover the tortilla with the tuna mixture.
4. After rolling, cut the tortilla in half.

Prep Time: 10 minutes Cook Time: None
- Nutritional Composition (per serving): -
  - 250 calories
  - 22g of protein
  - 12g of fat
  - 16g of carbohydrates
  - 2g of fiber

4. Avocado and Chicken Salad

Ingredients:
- 1/2 cup diced cooked chicken breast
- 1/2 diced ripe avocado
- 1/4 cup halved cherry tomatoes
- 1 tablespoon olive oil
- One teaspoon of lemon juice
- To taste, add salt and pepper.

Directions:
1. Put the chicken, avocado, and cherry tomatoes in a bowl.
2. Add a lemon juice and olive oil drizzle.
3. Add pepper and salt for seasoning.
4. Gently toss to mix.

Cook Time: None   Prep Time: 10 minutes
- Nutritional Composition (per serving):
  - 300 calories
  20g of protein
  - 20g of fat
  - 10g of carbohydrates
  - 6g of fiber

5. Roll-Ups with Cheese and Turkey

Ingredients:
- Two pieces of cheese (cheddar or Swiss)
- Four slices of deli turkey
- One whole wheat tortilla;
- One tablespoon Dijon mustard

Directions:
1. Spread the Dijon mustard over the tortilla and lay it flat.
2. Arrange cheese and turkey slices on the tortilla.
3. Tightly roll the tortilla.
4. Cut into pieces that are bite-sized.

Cook Time: None - Nutritional Composition (per serving): -
Prep Time: 5 minutes
- 280 calories
- 18g of protein
- 14g of fat
- 22g of carbohydrates
- 2g of fiber

6. Egg Muffins with Vegetables

Ingredients:
- Four eggs
- 1/4 cup sliced bell pepper
- 1/2 cup chopped spinach
- 1/4 cup shredded cheese
- To taste, add salt and pepper.

Directions:
1. Set oven temperature to 175°C/350°F.
2. Combine eggs, spinach, cheese, bell pepper, salt, and pepper in a bowl.
3. Fill muffin tin with mixture after greasing it.
4. Bake until firm, 20 to 25 minutes.

Cook Time: 25 minutes - Prep Time: 10 minutes
Nutritional Information (per two muffin serving):
- 200 calories
 14g of protein
- 14g of fat
- 3g of carbohydrates
- 1g of fiber

7. Creamy Soup with Spinach

Ingredients:
- 1/2 cup milk or a dairy substitute
- 1 cup low-sodium chicken broth
- 2 cups fresh spinach
- One small onion, chopped
- One small potato, peeled and diced
- One tablespoon olive oil
- To taste, add salt and pepper.

Directions:
1. In a pot over medium heat, warm the olive oil.
2. Add potato and onion and cook until tender.
3. Include chicken broth and heat until it boils.

4. Cook the spinach until it wilts.

5. Use a blender to puree the soup until it's smooth.

6. Add the milk and season with the pepper and salt.

Cook Time: 20 minutes - Prep Time: 10 minutes
- Nutritional Composition (per serving):
- 180 calories
- Six grams of protein
- 8g of fat
- 24g of carbohydrates
- 3g of fiber

8. Lemon-Baked Salmon

Ingredients:
- One 4-oz salmon fillet
- One tablespoon olive oil
- One tablespoon lemon juice
- To taste, add salt and pepper.

Directions:
1. Set oven temperature to 190°C/375°F.
2. Arrange the salmon on a baking tray.
3. Add a lemon juice and olive oil drizzle.
4. Add pepper and salt for seasoning.
5. Bake until cooked through, 15 to 20 minutes.

Cook Time: 20 minutes - Prep Time: 5 minutes
- Nutritional Composition (per serving):

- 250 calories, 23g of protein,   - 17g of fat
  - 0g of carbohydrates   - Fiber: 0 g

9. Leafy Green and Quinoa Salad

Ingredients:
- 1/4 cup sliced cucumber,
- 1/4 cup diced bell pepper,
- 1/2 cup cooked quinoa,
- 1/4 cup halved cherry tomatoes
- 1 tablespoon olive oil
- 1 teaspoon lemon juice
- To taste, add salt and pepper.

Directions:
1. Put the cooked quinoa, cucumber, cherry tomatoes, and bell pepper in a bowl.
2. Add a lemon juice and olive oil drizzle.
3. Add pepper and salt for seasoning.
4. Gently toss to mix.

Prep Time: 10 minutes Cook Time: None
Nutritional Composition (per serving):
- 220 calories
- Six grams of protein
- 10g of fat
- 28g of carbohydrates
- 5g of fiber

10. Pesto-Crusted Zucchini Noodles

Ingredients:
- Two medium-sized spiralized zucchini
- 1/4 cup of pesto.
- One tablespoon of olive oil
To taste, add salt and pepper.

Directions:
1. In a pan over medium heat, warm the olive oil.
2. When the zucchini noodles start to soften, add them and sauté for two to three minutes.
3. Take off the heat and combine with the pesto sauce.
4. Add pepper and salt for seasoning.

Cook Time: 5 minutes - Prep Time: 10 minutes
- Nutritional Composition (per serving):
   - 180 calories   - 3g of protein, 16g of fat, 7g of carbohydrates, and 2g of fiber

11. Avocado and Turkey Sandwich

Ingredients:
- Half a ripe avocado, sliced
- Four slices of deli turkey
- Two slices of whole grain bread
- One tablespoon mayonnaise
- One lettuce leaf

Directions:
1. On a single piece of bread, spread mayonnaise.
2. Arrange lettuce, turkey, and avocado slices in layers.
3. Place the second piece of bread on top.
4. Divide in half and present.

Cook Time: None Prep Time: 5 minutes
- Nutritional Composition (per serving): -
   - 300 calories
   - 18g of protein
   - 14g of fat
   - 30g of carbohydrates
   - 6g of fiber

12. Stir-fried chicken and veggies

Ingredients:
- 1/2 cup sliced cooked chicken breast
- 1/2 cup of florets of broccoli
- 1/2 cup chopped bell pepper
- 1/4 cup chopped carrot
- One tablespoon soy sauce
- One tablespoon olive oil
- One teaspoon (optional) sesame seeds

Directions:
1. In a pan over medium heat, warm the olive oil.
2. Sauté the carrot, bell pepper, and broccoli for five minutes.
3. Include the soy sauce and cooked chicken.

4. Cook for a further two to three minutes.
5. If preferred, top with sesame seeds.

Cook Time: 10 minutes
- Nutritional Composition (per serving):
    - 250 calories, 20g of protein, 10g of fat
    - 18g of carbohydrates
    - 5g of fiber

13. Carrot and Lentil Soup

Ingredients:
- 1/2 cup red lentils
- 1 chopped, peeled carrot
- 1 chopped tiny onion
- One teaspoon cumin
- One tablespoon olive oil
- Two cups low-sodium vegetable broth
- To taste, add salt and pepper.

Directions:
1. In a pot over medium heat, warm the olive oil.
2. Add the onion and carrot and cook until they become tender.
3. Include the cumin, lentils, and vegetable broth.
4. Bring to a boil, then simmer for 20 minutes on low heat.
5. Add pepper and salt for seasoning.

Cook Time: 25 minutes - Prep Time: 10 minutes
- Nutritional Composition (per serving): - 200 calories
12g of protein, - 5g of fat, - 30g of carbohydrates, 10g of fiber

14. Cracker Salad with Egg

Ingredients:
- 2 chopped cooked eggs
- 2 tablespoons mayonnaise
- One tsp mustard, six whole grain crackers, and salt and pepper to taste

Directions:
1. In a bowl, combine chopped eggs, mustard, mayonnaise, salt, and pepper.
2. Transfer egg salad to cracker slices.

Cook Time: None Prep Time: 5 minutes
- Nutritional Composition (per serving):
  - 250 calories
  - 10g of protein
  - 18g of fat
  - 14g of carbohydrates
  - 3g of fiber

15. Avocado and Shrimp Salad

Ingredients:
- 1/2 cup cooked shrimp
- 1/2 diced ripe avocado
- 1/4 cup halved cherry tomatoes
- 1 tablespoon olive oil
- One teaspoon of lemon juice
- To taste, add salt and pepper.

Directions:
1. Put the shrimp, avocado, and cherry tomatoes in a bowl.
2. Add a lemon juice and olive oil drizzle.
3. Add pepper and salt for seasoning.
4. Gently toss to mix.

Cook Time: None - Prep Time: 10 minutes
- Nutritional Composition (per serving):
  - 220 calories
  - 15g of protein
  - 14g of fat
  - 8g of carbohydrates
  - 4g of fiber

Chapter 6: Dinner Recipes

15 Dinner Recipes for a Gastroparesis Diet for Seniors

1. Baked Chicken with Sweet Potatoes

Ingredients:
- 1 chicken breast (4 oz)
- 1 medium sweet potato, peeled and diced
- 1 tbsp olive oil
- 1 tsp paprika
- Salt and pepper to taste

Instructions:
1. Preheat oven to 375°F (190°C).
2. Toss sweet potato with olive oil, paprika, salt, and pepper.
3. Place diced sweet potato on a baking sheet.
4. Season chicken breast with salt and pepper.
5. Place chicken breast on the baking sheet with sweet potatoes.
6. Bake for 25-30 minutes or until chicken is cooked through and sweet potatoes are tender.

- Prep Time: 10 minutes- Cook Time: 30 minutes
- Nutritional Composition (per serving):
  - Calories: 280
  - Protein: 26g
  - Fat: 10g
  - Carbohydrates: 25g
  - Fiber: 4g

2. Creamy Chicken and Spinach Pasta

Ingredients:
- 1 cup cooked pasta
- 1/2 cup cooked chicken breast, diced
- 1 cup baby spinach
- 1/2 cup low-fat cream
- 1 tbsp olive oil
- 1/4 cup grated Parmesan cheese
- Salt and pepper to taste

Instructions:
1. Heat olive oil in a pan over medium heat.
2. Add chicken and spinach, cook until spinach is wilted.
3. Stir in cream and bring to a simmer.
4. Add cooked pasta and Parmesan cheese.
5. Season with salt and pepper.

- Prep Time: 10 minutes
- Cook Time: 10 minutes
- Nutritional Composition (per serving):
  - Calories: 320
  - Protein: 20g
  - Fat: 14g
  - Carbohydrates: 30g
  - Fiber: 3g

3. Salmon with Asparagus

Ingredients:
- 1 salmon fillet (4 oz)
- 1 cup asparagus spears
- 1 tbsp olive oil
- 1 tsp lemon zest
- Salt and pepper to taste

Instructions:
1. Preheat oven to 375°F (190°C).
2. Place salmon and asparagus on a baking sheet.
3. Drizzle with olive oil and sprinkle with lemon zest.
4. Season with salt and pepper.
5. Bake for 15-20 minutes or until salmon is cooked through and asparagus is tender.

- Prep Time: 5 minutes
- Cook Time: 20 minutes
- Nutritional Composition (per serving):
  - Calories: 260
  - Protein: 23g
  - Fat: 16g
  - Carbohydrates: 8g
  - Fiber: 4g

4. Turkey Meatballs with Mashed Cauliflower

Ingredients:
- 1/2 lb ground turkey
- 1/4 cup breadcrumbs
- 1 egg
- 1/4 cup finely chopped parsley
- 1/4 tsp garlic powder
- Salt and pepper to taste
- 1 head cauliflower, chopped
- 1/4 cup low-fat milk or milk alternative

Instructions:
1. Preheat oven to 375°F (190°C).
2. Mix ground turkey, breadcrumbs, egg, parsley, garlic powder, salt, and pepper in a bowl.
3. Form mixture into meatballs and place on a baking sheet.
4. Bake for 20 minutes or until cooked through.
5. Steam cauliflower until tender.
6. Mash cauliflower with milk and season with salt and pepper.

- Prep Time: 15 minutes
- Cook Time: 25 minutes
- Nutritional Composition (per serving):
  - Calories: 280
  - Protein: 22g
  - Fat: 12g
  - Carbohydrates: 20g

- Fiber: 6g

5. Stuffed Bell Peppers

Ingredients:
- 2 bell peppers, halved and seeded
- 1/2 cup cooked quinoa
- 1/2 cup ground turkey
- 1/4 cup diced tomatoes
- 1/4 cup shredded cheese
- 1 tbsp olive oil
- Salt and pepper to taste

Instructions:
1. Preheat oven to 375°F (190°C).
2. Heat olive oil in a pan and cook ground turkey until browned.
3. Mix in cooked quinoa and diced tomatoes.
4. Stuff bell pepper halves with the mixture.
5. Top with shredded cheese.
6. Place stuffed peppers on a baking sheet and bake for 25 minutes.

- Prep Time: 10 minutes
- Cook Time: 25 minutes
- Nutritional Composition (per serving):
  - Calories: 290
  - Protein: 20g
  - Fat: 14g
  - Carbohydrates: 20g
  - Fiber: 4g

6. Baked Cod with Carrots

Ingredients:
- 1 cod fillet (4 oz)
- 1 cup baby carrots
- 1 tbsp olive oil
- 1 tsp dried thyme
- Salt and pepper to taste

Instructions:
1. Preheat oven to 375°F (190°C).
2. Place cod fillet and carrots on a baking sheet.
3. Drizzle with olive oil and sprinkle with dried thyme.
4. Season with salt and pepper.
5. Bake for 15-20 minutes or until cod is cooked through and carrots are tender.

- Prep Time: 5 minutes
- Cook Time: 20 minutes
- Nutritional Composition (per serving):
  - Calories: 220
  - Protein: 22g
  - Fat: 12g
  - Carbohydrates: 10g
  - Fiber: 3g

7. Chicken and Broccoli Stir-Fry

Ingredients:
- 1/2 cup cooked chicken breast, sliced
- 1 cup broccoli florets
- 1/4 cup low-sodium chicken broth
- 1 tbsp soy sauce
- 1 tbsp olive oil
- 1 tsp cornstarch (optional, for thickening)

Instructions:
1. Heat olive oil in a pan over medium heat.
2. Add broccoli and cook until tender.
3. Add cooked chicken and chicken broth.
4. Stir in soy sauce and cornstarch if using.
5. Cook until sauce has thickened and chicken is heated through.

- Prep Time: 10 minutes
- Cook Time: 10 minutes
- Nutritional Composition (per serving):
  - Calories: 250
  - Protein: 20g
  - Fat: 10g
  - Carbohydrates: 20g
  - Fiber: 5g

8. Creamy Butternut Squash Soup

Ingredients:
- 2 cups diced butternut squash
- 1 cup low-sodium chicken broth
- 1/2 cup low-fat cream
- 1 small onion, diced
- 1 tbsp olive oil
- 1/4 tsp ground nutmeg
- Salt and pepper to taste

Instructions:
1. Heat olive oil in a pot over medium heat.
2. Add onion and cook until softened.
3. Add butternut squash and chicken broth.
4. Simmer until squash is tender.
5. Puree the soup using a blender until smooth.
6. Stir in cream and nutmeg.
7. Season with salt and pepper.

- Prep Time: 10 minutes
- Cook Time: 20 minutes
- Nutritional Composition (per serving):
  - Calories: 210
  - Protein: 4g
  - Fat: 12g
  - Carbohydrates: 26g
  - Fiber: 4g

9. Turkey and Spinach Stuffed Mushrooms

Ingredients:
- 6 large mushrooms, stems removed
- 1/2 cup ground turkey
- 1/4 cup chopped spinach
- 1/4 cup breadcrumbs
- 1 tbsp olive oil
- 1/4 cup shredded cheese

Instructions:
1. Preheat oven to 375°F (190°C).
2. Heat olive oil in a pan and cook ground turkey until browned.
3. Mix in spinach and breadcrumbs.
4. Stuff mushrooms with the mixture.
5. Top with shredded cheese.
6. Bake for 20 minutes or until mushrooms are tender.

- Prep Time: 15 minutes
- Cook Time: 20 minutes
- Nutritional Composition (per serving):
  - Calories: 240
  - Protein: 18g
  - Fat: 14g
  - Carbohydrates: 14g
  - Fiber: 3g

10. Shrimp and Rice Skillet

Ingredients:
- 1/2 cup cooked shrimp
- 1/2 cup cooked white rice
- 1/2 cup diced bell pepper
- 1/4 cup low-sodium chicken broth
- 1 tbsp olive oil
- Salt and pepper to taste

Instructions:
1. Heat olive oil in a skillet over medium heat.
2. Add bell pepper and cook until softened.
3. Stir in cooked shrimp and chicken broth.
4. Add cooked rice and stir until heated through.
5. Season with salt and pepper.

- Prep Time: 10 minutes
- Cook Time: 10 minutes
- Nutritional Composition (per serving):
  - Calories: 280
  - Protein: 18g
  - Fat: 10g
  - Carbohydrates: 30g
  - Fiber: 2g

11. Baked Tilapia with Green Beans

Ingredients:
- 1 tilapia fillet (4 oz)
- 1 cup green beans
- 1 tbsp olive oil
- 1 tsp dried dill
- Salt and pepper to taste

Instructions:
1. Preheat oven to 375°F (190°C).
2. Place tilapia fillet and green beans on a baking sheet.
3. Drizzle with olive oil and sprinkle with dried dill.
4. Season with salt and pepper.
5. Bake for 15-20 minutes or until tilapia is cooked through and green beans are tender.

- Prep Time: 5 minutes
- Cook Time: 20 minutes
- Nutritional Composition (per serving):
  - Calories: 220
  - Protein: 23g
  - Fat: 10g
  - Carbohydrates: 12g
  - Fiber: 4g

12. Chicken and Sweet Potato Curry

Ingredients:
- 1/2 cup cooked chicken breast, diced
- 1 medium sweet potato, peeled and cubed
- 1/2 cup light coconut milk
- 1 tbsp curry powder
- 1 tbsp olive oil
- Salt to taste

Instructions:
1. Heat olive oil in a pan over medium heat.
2. Add sweet potato and cook until starting to soften.
3. Stir in curry powder and cook for 1 minute.
4. Add chicken and coconut milk.
5. Simmer until sweet potato is tender and chicken is heated through.
6. Season with salt.

- Prep Time: 10 minutes
- Cook Time: 20 minutes
- Nutritional Composition (per serving):
  - Calories: 280
  - Protein: 20g
  - Fat: 12g
  - Carbohydrates: 28g
  - Fiber: 4g

13. Spinach and Cheese Stuffed Chicken

Ingredients:
- 1 chicken breast (4 oz)
- 1/2 cup chopped spinach
- 1/4 cup shredded cheese
- 1 tbsp olive oil
- Salt and pepper to taste

Instructions:
1. Preheat oven to 375°F (190°C).
2. Carefully cut a pocket into the chicken breast.
3. Stuff with spinach and cheese.
4. Secure with toothpicks if needed.
5. Season with salt and pepper.
6. Heat olive oil in a skillet over medium heat.
7. Sear chicken on both sides until golden.
8. Transfer to the oven and bake for 20 minutes or until cooked through.

- Prep Time: 10 minutes
- Cook Time: 30 minutes
- Nutritional Composition (per serving):
  - Calories: 290
  - Protein: 30g
  - Fat: 16g
  - Carbohydrates: 6g
  - Fiber: 2g

14. Creamy Zucchini and Tomato Bake

Ingredients:
- 1 zucchini, sliced
- 1 cup cherry tomatoes, halved
- 1/2 cup low-fat cream
- 1/4 cup grated Parmesan cheese
- 1 tbsp olive oil
- Salt and pepper to taste

Instructions:
1. Preheat oven to 375°F (190°C).
2. Layer zucchini and cherry tomatoes in a baking dish.
3. Drizzle with olive oil and season with salt and pepper.
4. Pour cream over vegetables.
5. Sprinkle with Parmesan cheese.
6. Bake for 25 minutes or until vegetables are tender and cheese is golden.

- Prep Time: 10 minutes
- Cook Time: 25 minutes
- Nutritional Composition (per serving):
  - Calories: 230
  - Protein: 8g
  - Fat: 16g
  - Carbohydrates: 16g
  - Fiber: 4g

15. Beef and Vegetable Stir-Fry

Ingredients:
- 1/2 cup cooked beef strips
- 1/2 cup bell pepper, sliced
- 1/2 cup snow peas
- 1/4 cup low-sodium beef broth
- 1 tbsp soy sauce
- 1 tbsp olive oil

Instructions:
1. Heat olive oil in a pan over medium heat.
2. Add bell pepper and snow peas, cook until tender.
3. Add cooked beef and beef broth.
4. Stir in soy sauce and cook until heated through.

- Prep Time: 10 minutes
- Cook Time: 10 minutes
- Nutritional Composition (per serving):
  - Calories: 290
  - Protein: 22g
  - Fat: 15g
  - Carbohydrates: 14g
  - Fiber: 4g

These recipes are designed to be gentle on the digestive system while providing balanced nutrition suitable for seniors managing gastroparesis.

Chapter 7: Snack Recipes

10 Snack Recipes for an Older Adult Gastroparesis Diet

1. Honey-Berry Greek Yogurt

Ingredients:
- One cup of Greek yogurt
- 1/2 cup mixed berries (strawberries, blueberries, raspberries)
- 1 tablespoon honey

Directions:
1. Place a portion of Greek yogurt in a bowl.
2. Drizzle yogurt with honey.
3. Place mixed berries on top.

Cook Time: None - Prep Time: 5 minutes

- Nutritional Composition (per serving): - 200 calories
  12g of protein, 4g of fat, 30g of carbohydrates, 4g of fiber

2. Banana and Smooth Peanut Butter

Ingredients:
- One sliced banana
- Two tsp of creamy peanut butter

Directions:
1. Cut the banana into slices.
2. Apply peanut butter to every piece.

Cook Time: None - Prep Time: 5 minutes

Nutritional Composition (per serving): - 250 calories, Six grams of protein, 16g of fat, 24g of carbohydrates, 3g of fiber

3. Pineapple and Cottage Cheese

Ingredients:
- 1/2 cup of cottage cheese
- 1/2 cup of canned or fresh pineapple chunks

Directions:
1. Place a portion of cottage cheese in a bowl.
2. Add pineapple slices on top.

Cook Time: None - Prep Time: 5 minutes
- Nutritional Composition (per serving): - 140 calories
  - 14g of protein, - 3g of fat - 15g of carbohydrates
  - 1g of fiber

4. Cucumber slices with hummus

Ingredients:
- 1/4 cup hummus - 1 sliced cucumber

Directions:
1. Transfer the hummus to a little bowl.
2. Cut the cucumber into rounds.
3. Present cucumber slices for dipping with hummus.

Cook Time: None - Prep Time: 5 minutes
Nutritional Composition (per serving): - 120 calories
  - 4g of protein

- 6g of fat
- 14g of carbohydrates
- 4g of fiber

5. Cinnamon Applesauce

Ingredients:
- One cup of plain applesauce
- Half a teaspoon of ground cinnamon

Directions:
1. First, transfer applesauce to a bowl.
2. Add some ground cinnamon there.

Cook Time: None - Prep Time: 2 minutes
Nutritional Composition (per serving): - 100 calories
  - Protein: 0 grams
  - Fat: 0 g
  - 25g of carbohydrates
  - 3g of fiber

6. Avocado and Rice Cakes

Ingredients:
- Two cakes of ordinary rice
- 1/2 mashed, ripe avocado
- To taste, add salt and pepper.

Directions:
1. Top each rice cake with mashed avocado.
2. Add pepper and salt for seasoning.

Cook Time: None - Prep Time: 5 minutes

Nutritional Composition (per serving): - 160 calories
- 2g of protein   - 10g of fat   - 15g of carbohydrates
- 5g of fiber

7. Cheese with Grapes

Ingredients:
- One ounce of cubed cheddar cheese
- 1/2 cup grapes without seeds

Directions:
1. Cut cheddar cheese into cubes.
2. Accompany with unseeded grapes.

Cook Time: None - Prep Time: 5 minutes
Nutritional Composition (per serving): - 200 calories
- 8g of protein
- 14g of fat
- 12g of carbohydrates
- 1g of fiber

8. Cheddar Egg

Ingredients:
- One egg

Directions:
1. Put the egg in a pan with water on top.
2. Bring to a boil, then simmer for ten minutes on low heat.
3. Take out of the water, allow to cool, peel, and savor.

Cook Time: 10 minutes - Prep Time: 5 minutes
Nutritional Composition (per serving): - 70 calories

- Six grams of protein   - 5g of fat
- 1g of carbohydrates
- Fiber: 0 g

9. Dried Cranberries and Almonds

Ingredients:
 − 1/4 cup almonds
 − 1/4 cup of cranberries, dried

Directions:
 1. In a small bowl, combine almonds and dried cranberries.

Cook Time: None - Prep Time: 2 minutes
- Nutritional Composition (per serving): - 200 calories
  - 5g of protein   - 12g of fat   - 20g of carbohydrates
  - 3g of fiber

10. Apple Chips Baked

Ingredients:
 Two finely sliced apples and half a teaspoon of ground cinnamon
Directions:
 1. Set oven temperature to 200°F, or 95°C.
 2. Place apple slices in an arrangement on a parchment paper-lined baking sheet.
 3. Add a dash of ground cinnamon.
 4. Bake until crisp, turning halfway during the two hours of baking.

Cook Time: 2 hours - Prep Time: 10 minutes

Nutritional Composition (per serving): - 100 calories
  - Protein: 0 grams   - Fat: 0 g   - 26g of carbohydrates
  - 5g of fiber

Chapter 8: Nutritious Desserts

10 Dessert Recipes for a Gastroparesis Diet

1. Banana Soft Serve

Ingredients:
  - 2 ripe bananas, sliced and frozen
  - 1 tsp vanilla extract

Instructions:
  1. Place frozen banana slices in a blender.
  2. Add vanilla extract.
  3. Blend until smooth and creamy.
  4. Serve immediately.

- Prep Time: 5 minutes
- Cook Time: None
- Nutritional Composition (per serving):
  - Calories: 105
  - Protein: 1g
  - Fat: 0g
  - Carbohydrates: 27g
  - Fiber: 3g

2. Applesauce Gelatin

Ingredients:
- 1 cup unsweetened applesauce
- 1 packet unflavored gelatin
- 1/4 cup water
- 1 tsp cinnamon

Instructions:
1. In a small saucepan, sprinkle gelatin over water and let it sit for 1 minute.
2. Heat over low heat, stirring until gelatin dissolves.
3. Remove from heat and stir in applesauce and cinnamon.
4. Pour into molds and refrigerate until set, about 2 hours.

- Prep Time: 10 minutes
- Cook Time: 2 hours (chilling time)
- Nutritional Composition (per serving):
  - Calories: 70
  - Protein: 1g
  - Fat: 0g
  - Carbohydrates: 17g
  - Fiber: 2g

3. Yogurt and Berry Parfait

Ingredients:
- 1 cup Greek yogurt
- 1/2 cup mixed berries
- 1 tbsp honey

Instructions:
1. Layer Greek yogurt, mixed berries, and honey in a glass or bowl.
2. Repeat layers until all ingredients are used.
3. Serve immediately.

- Prep Time: 5 minutes
- Cook Time: None
- Nutritional Composition (per serving):
  - Calories: 160
  - Protein: 10g
  - Fat: 2g
  - Carbohydrates: 30g
  - Fiber: 3g

4. Chia Pudding

Ingredients:
- 1 cup almond milk
- 1/4 cup chia seeds
- 1 tbsp maple syrup
- 1/2 tsp vanilla extract

Instructions:
1. In a bowl, mix almond milk, chia seeds, maple syrup, and vanilla extract.
2. Stir well to combine.
3. Refrigerate for at least 2 hours or overnight until thickened.

- Prep Time: 5 minutes
- Cook Time: 2 hours (chilling time)
- Nutritional Composition (per serving):
  - Calories: 140
  - Protein: 4g
  - Fat: 7g
  - Carbohydrates: 17g
  - Fiber: 10g

5. Baked Pears with Honey

Ingredients:
- 2 pears, halved and cored
- 2 tbsp honey
- 1/2 tsp ground cinnamon

Instructions:
1. Preheat oven to 350°F (175°C).
2. Place pear halves in a baking dish.
3. Drizzle with honey and sprinkle with cinnamon.
4. Bake for 20 minutes or until tender.

- Prep Time: 5 minutes   - Cook Time: 20 minutes
- Nutritional Composition (per serving):   - Calories: 140
  - Protein: 1g   - Fat: 0g   - Carbohydrates: 36g
  - Fiber: 6g

6. Rice Pudding

Ingredients:
- 1 cup cooked white rice
- 1 cup low-fat milk
- 2 tbsp sugar
- 1/2 tsp vanilla extract
- 1/4 tsp ground cinnamon

Instructions:
1. In a saucepan, combine cooked rice, milk, sugar, and vanilla extract.
2. Cook over medium heat, stirring frequently, until thickened, about 20 minutes.
3. Sprinkle with cinnamon before serving.

- Prep Time: 5 minutes   - Cook Time: 20 minutes
- Nutritional Composition (per serving):   - Calories: 180
  - Protein: 4g - Fat: 2g   - Carbohydrates: 36g - Fiber: 1g

7. Mango Sorbet

Ingredients:
- 2 ripe mangoes, peeled and chopped
- 1 tbsp lime juice
- 1 tbsp honey

Instructions:
1. Freeze chopped mangoes for at least 4 hours.
2. In a blender, combine frozen mangoes, lime juice, and honey.
3. Blend until smooth and creamy.
4. Serve immediately.

- Prep Time: 10 minutes
- Cook Time: 4 hours (freezing time)
- Nutritional Composition (per serving):
  - Calories: 130
  - Protein: 1g
  - Fat: 0g
  - Carbohydrates: 34g
  - Fiber: 3g

8. Vanilla Pudding

Ingredients:
- 2 cups low-fat milk
- 1/4 cup sugar
- 3 tbsp cornstarch
- 1 tsp vanilla extract

Instructions:
1. In a saucepan, combine milk, sugar, and cornstarch.
2. Cook over medium heat, stirring constantly, until thickened, about 10 minutes.
3. Remove from heat and stir in vanilla extract.
4. Pour into serving dishes and refrigerate until set, about 2 hours.

- Prep Time: 5 minutes
- Cook Time: 10 minutes + 2 hours (chilling time)
- Nutritional Composition (per serving):
  - Calories: 130
  - Protein: 4g
  - Fat: 2g
  - Carbohydrates: 26g
  - Fiber: 0g

9. Strawberry Banana Smoothie

Ingredients:
- 1 cup strawberries, hulled
- 1 banana
- 1 cup low-fat yogurt
- 1/2 cup almond milk

Instructions:
1. In a blender, combine strawberries, banana, yogurt, and almond milk.
2. Blend until smooth.
3. Serve immediately.

- Prep Time: 5 minutes   - Cook Time: None
- Nutritional Composition (per serving):
  - Calories: 180
  - Protein: 6g
  - Fat: 2g
  - Carbohydrates: 36g
  - Fiber: 4g

10. Blueberry Muffins

Ingredients:
- 1 cup flour
- 1/2 cup sugar
- 1 tsp baking powder
- 1/2 tsp baking soda
- 1/4 tsp salt
- 1/2 cup low-fat yogurt
- 1/4 cup milk
- 1 egg
- 1/4 cup vegetable oil
- 1 cup blueberries

Instructions:
1. Preheat oven to 375°F (190°C).
2. In a bowl, combine flour, sugar, baking powder, baking soda, and salt.
3. In another bowl, whisk together yogurt, milk, egg, and vegetable oil.
4. Add wet ingredients to dry ingredients and stir until just combined.
5. Fold in blueberries.
6. Spoon batter into a greased muffin tin.
7. Bake for 20-25 minutes or until a toothpick inserted into the center comes out clean.

- Prep Time: 10 minutes   - Cook Time: 20-25 minutes
- Nutritional Composition (per serving, based on 12 muffins):
  - Calories: 150   - Protein: 3g   - Fat: 6g
  - Carbohydrates: 22g   - Fiber: 1g

Chapter 9: Healthy Beverages

15 Beverage Recipes for a Gastroparesis Diet for Seniors

1. Banana Almond Smoothie

Ingredients:
- 1 banana
- 1 cup almond milk
- 1 tbsp almond butter
- 1 tsp honey (optional)

Instructions:
1. Blend banana, almond milk, almond butter, and honey until smooth.
2. Serve immediately.

- Prep Time: 5 minutes
- Cook Time: None
- Nutritional Composition (per serving):
  - Calories: 180
  - Protein: 3g
  - Fat: 7g
  - Carbohydrates: 27g
  - Fiber: 3g

2. Peach Ginger Smoothie

Ingredients:
- 1 cup frozen peaches
- 1/2 inch piece fresh ginger, peeled and grated
- 1 cup low-fat yogurt
- 1/2 cup water

Instructions:
1. Blend peaches, ginger, yogurt, and water until smooth.
2. Serve immediately.

- Prep Time: 5 minutes   - Cook Time: None
- Nutritional Composition (per serving): - Calories: 150
  - Protein: 6g - Fat: 2g - Carbohydrates: 28g   - Fiber: 2g

3. Cucumber Mint Cooler

Ingredients:
- 1 cucumber, peeled and sliced
- 1 tbsp fresh mint leaves
- 1 cup water
- 1 tsp honey (optional)

Instructions:
1. Blend cucumber, mint leaves, water, and honey until smooth.
2. Strain if desired and serve immediately.

- Prep Time: 5 minutes   - Cook Time: None
- Nutritional Composition (per serving): - Calories: 30
  - Protein: 1g - Fat: 0g - Carbohydrates: 8g - Fiber: 1g

4. Berry Kefir Smoothie

Ingredients:
- 1 cup mixed berries (strawberries, blueberries, raspberries)
- 1 cup kefir
- 1 tsp honey (optional)

Instructions:
1. Blend mixed berries, kefir, and honey until smooth.
2. Serve immediately.

- Prep Time: 5 minutes   - Cook Time: None
- Nutritional Composition (per serving):   - Calories: 130
  - Protein: 6g - Fat: 3g - Carbohydrates: 22g - Fiber: 4g

5. Mango Lassi

Ingredients:
- 1 cup mango, chopped
- 1 cup low-fat yogurt
- 1/2 cup water
- 1 tsp honey (optional)

Instructions:
1. Blend mango, yogurt, water, and honey until smooth.
2. Serve immediately.

- Prep Time: 5 minutes   - Cook Time: None
- Nutritional Composition (per serving):   - Calories: 160
  - Protein: 6g - Fat: 2g - Carbohydrates: 30g - Fiber: 2g

6. Pineapple Coconut Water

Ingredients:
- 1 cup pineapple, chopped
- 1 cup coconut water

Instructions:
1. Blend pineapple and coconut water until smooth.
2. Serve immediately.

- Prep Time: 5 minutes   - Cook Time: None
- Nutritional Composition (per serving):   - Calories: 70
  - Protein: 0g - Fat: 0g - Carbohydrates: 18g - Fiber: 2g

7. Carrot Orange Juice

Ingredients:
- 1 cup carrot juice
- 1 cup orange juice

Instructions:
1. Mix carrot juice and orange juice.
2. Serve immediately.

- Prep Time: 5 minutes   - Cook Time: None
- Nutritional Composition (per serving): - Calories: 110
  - Protein: 2g - Fat: 0g - Carbohydrates: 27g - Fiber: 2g

8. Apple Cinnamon Water

Ingredients:
- 1 apple, sliced
- 1 cinnamon stick
- 1 liter water

Instructions:
1. Add apple slices and cinnamon stick to water.
2. Refrigerate for at least 1 hour before serving.

- Prep Time: 5 minutes - Cook Time: 1 hour (infusion time)
- Nutritional Composition (per serving): - Calories: 5
  - Protein: 0g - Fat: 0g - Carbohydrates: 1g   - Fiber: 0g

9. Blueberry Lemonade

Ingredients:
- 1 cup blueberries
- 1/2 cup lemon juice
- 1 tbsp honey
- 2 cups water

Instructions:
1. Blend blueberries, lemon juice, honey, and water until smooth.
2. Strain if desired and serve immediately.

- Prep Time: 5 minutes- Cook Time: None
- Nutritional Composition (per serving):   - Calories: 60
  - Protein: 0g - Fat: 0g - Carbohydrates: 15g - Fiber: 2g

10. Watermelon Mint Smoothie

Ingredients:
- 2 cups watermelon, chopped
- 1 tbsp fresh mint leaves
- 1 cup water

Instructions:
1. Blend watermelon, mint leaves, and water until smooth.
2. Serve immediately.

- Prep Time: 5 minutes   - Cook Time: None
- Nutritional Composition (per serving): - Calories: 50
  - Protein: 1g - Fat: 0g - Carbohydrates: 12g - Fiber: 1g

11. Papaya Lime Smoothie

Ingredients:
- 1 cup papaya, chopped
- 1 cup low-fat yogurt
- 1 tbsp lime juice

Instructions:
1. Blend papaya, yogurt, and lime juice until smooth.
2. Serve immediately.

- Prep Time: 5 minutes - Cook Time: None
- Nutritional Composition (per serving):   - Calories: 110
  - Protein: 6g - Fat: 2g - Carbohydrates: 20g - Fiber: 3g

12. Strawberry Basil Infused Water

Ingredients:
- 1 cup strawberries, sliced
- 1/4 cup fresh basil leaves
- 1 liter water

Instructions:
1. Add strawberries and basil leaves to water.
2. Refrigerate for at least 1 hour before serving.

- Prep Time: 5 minutes - Cook Time: 1 hour (infusion time)
- Nutritional Composition (per serving): - Calories: 5
  - Protein: 0g - Fat: 0g - Carbohydrates: 1g - Fiber: 0g

13. Ginger Lemon Tea

Ingredients:
- 1 cup water
- 1-inch piece fresh ginger, peeled and sliced
- 1 tbsp lemon juice
- 1 tsp honey (optional)

Instructions:
1. Boil water with ginger slices for 10 minutes.
2. Remove ginger slices and add lemon juice and honey.
3. Serve warm.

- Prep Time: 5 minutes   - Cook Time: 10 minutes
- Nutritional Composition (per serving): - Calories: 20
  - Protein: 0g - Fat: 0g - Carbohydrates: 5g - Fiber: 0g

14. Pear Vanilla Smoothie

Ingredients:
- 1 pear, peeled and chopped
- 1 cup low-fat milk
- 1/2 tsp vanilla extract
- 1 tsp honey (optional)

Instructions:

1. Blend pear, milk, vanilla extract, and honey until smooth.

2. Serve immediately.

- Prep Time: 5 minutes
- Cook Time: None
- Nutritional Composition (per serving):
  - Calories: 120
  - Protein: 5g
  - Fat: 2g
  - Carbohydrates: 22g
  - Fiber: 3g

15. Coconut Mango Smoothie

Ingredients:
- 1 cup mango, chopped
- 1 cup coconut milk
- 1 tsp honey (optional)

Instructions:
1. Blend mango, coconut milk, and honey until smooth.
2. Serve immediately.

- Prep Time: 5 minutes
- Cook Time: None
- Nutritional Composition (per serving):
  - Calories: 180
  - Protein: 1g
  - Fat: 11g
  - Carbohydrates: 21g
  - Fiber: 2g

These beverage recipes are designed to be gentle on the digestive system, providing hydration and essential nutrients while catering to the dietary needs of seniors managing gastroparesis.

Chapter 10: Particular Dietary Requirements

Recognizing Personal Needs

It's critical to understand that every person's experience with gastroparesis varies greatly when it comes to management. A person's nutritional needs, underlying medical issues, and the intensity of their symptoms are all important considerations for figuring out the best course of action. This chapter explores the particular dietary considerations that must be made in order to manage gastroparesis efficiently and enhance the quality of life for older adults.

Juggling Nutritional Requirements

It can be difficult to maintain proper diet when treating gastroparesis. Maintaining a balanced diet with enough calories, protein, vitamins, and minerals is the major objective. Considering the small range of foods that may be tolerated, it's critical to concentrate on nutrient-dense choices. For example, nutritional supplements and liquid meals can be helpful in supplying essential nutrients without putting too much strain on the digestive system. Having a dietitian's advice can be quite helpful in coming up with a meal plan that suits each person's nutritional requirements.

Protein-Related Considerations

Maintaining muscle mass and general health requires protein, but eating enough of it can be challenging while suffering from gastroparesis. Protein foods that are soft and simple to digest, such yogurt, tofu, and eggs, are frequently more well-tolerated. Adding protein powders to drinks and smoothies can also increase the amount of protein consumed. To make sure the person is getting the nutrients they need without aggravating their symptoms, it's critical to keep an eye on their tolerance to various protein sources and make adjustments as necessary.

Handling Intake of Fiber

Although fiber is essential to a balanced diet, people with gastroparesis may find it difficult to consume it. Raw or uncooked foods that are high in fiber might be difficult to digest and exacerbate symptoms. However, since fiber is essential for digestive health, doing away with it entirely is not advised. Soluble fiber, which is found in foods like oatmeal, bananas, and cooked vegetables and is easier to digest, should be the main focus. Small doses of soluble fiber added gradually while keeping an eye on tolerance can help preserve digestive health without producing discomfort.

Considerations for Fat Intake

For those who have gastroparesis, slowing stomach emptying is a major worry due to the potential effects of fat. Nonetheless, since they maintain cell activity and provide energy, fats are a necessary component of a balanced diet. Moderation in the selection and consumption of healthy fats is crucial. Nut butters, avocados, and olive oil are good sources of good fats. Small, sensible servings of these fats can help guarantee sufficient consumption without aggravating symptoms. Individual tolerance varies, therefore it's important to keep an eye on how each person responds to different forms of fat and modify the diet accordingly.

Hydration

Particularly for seniors who may already be at risk for dehydration, staying hydrated is crucial. Hydration problems resulting from gastroparesis may include symptoms such as nausea and vomiting. Drinking small amounts of water throughout the day as opposed to a large one can help you stay hydrated without turning your stomach. Oral rehydration treatments and sports drinks, which are high in electrolytes, can also be helpful. It is essential for general health and wellbeing to keep an eye on one's level of hydration and to take immediate action when dehydration is detected.

Dealing with Weight Control

For seniors with gastroparesis, weight control can be a major worry. Unintentional weight loss is frequently brought on by decreased appetite and trouble with food digestion. However, some people may experience weight gain if they depend on meals high in calories but poor in nutrients to treat their symptoms. It's crucial to collaborate with a dietician or healthcare professional to create a customized eating plan that promotes healthy weight maintenance. Foods and supplements that are high in nutrients and readily absorbed can help guarantee a sufficient intake of calories without sacrificing the quality of the nutrients.

Time and Frequency of Meals

It might not be appropriate for people with gastroparesis to follow standard meal schedules. By keeping the stomach from getting overly full, eating smaller, more frequent meals throughout the day can help manage symptoms. This strategy can also aid in guaranteeing a consistent consumption of calories and nutrients. Setting aside time for meals and snacks can help seniors stay on track with their routines, which can help with symptom management and better digestion in general.

Handling Conditions That Already Exist

When designing their diet, seniors with gastroparesis frequently have other medical issues to take into account. Health issues like diabetes, heart disease, and hypertension can affect food choices and need to be carefully managed. For example, a diabetic may need to monitor their carbohydrate consumption closely, while a heart patient may need to reduce their intake of sodium and dangerous fats. Developing a food plan that promotes overall health requires coordinating care with healthcare experts to address all health issues holistically.

Adding to the Diet

Supplements to the diet could be required in some situations to guarantee sufficient consumption of nutrients. Supplements containing multivitamins, calcium, vitamin D, and iron can help close any nutritional gaps that may result from following a restricted diet. To guarantee they are suitable for the patient's needs and to prevent possible drug interactions, supplements should only be taken under a doctor's supervision.

Social and Psychological Aspects

It might be difficult to manage gastroparesis emotionally, socially, and physically. Eating is frequently a social activity, and going out to eat and social events can be difficult due to dietary limitations. It's critical to address these issues and discover strategies for enjoying meals and social gatherings. Whether in-person or virtual, joining support groups can foster a feeling of camaraderie and mutual understanding. Getting therapy or counseling can also help you handle the emotional effects of having a chronic illness.

Customizing Your Diet

In the end, a gastroparesis diet that is customized to a person's unique requirements and tastes is the most beneficial one. Since symptoms and tolerances might vary over time, this calls for constant observation and modification. Better nutritional planning is possible by keeping a food journal, which can be used to document which foods are well-tolerated and which ones create problems. Dietitians and medical professionals can be consulted on a regular basis to make sure the diet is still supporting general health and meeting nutritional demands.

Geriatric gastroparesis management necessitates a personalized and sophisticated strategy. Seniors can preserve their health and enhance their quality of life by concentrating on nutrient-dense foods, controlling their intake of fiber and fat, drinking plenty of water, and taking care of any co-existing diseases. It's critical to acknowledge the psychological and social difficulties associated with having gastroparesis and to get help when required. You may design a diet that promotes overall wellbeing and digestive health with careful planning and expert coaching.

Chapter11: Gastroparesis Management Through Lifestyle Changes

Living with gastroparesis means managing symptoms and preserving a high quality of life demands a comprehensive strategy, not just dietary changes. This chapter provides helpful lifestyle suggestions to assist seniors properly manage their gastroparesis and live a more pleasant and meaningful life.

Patterns and Habits of Eating

Modifying eating habits and patterns is a crucial aspect of controlling gastroparesis through lifestyle changes. The following are some crucial tactics:

1. Small, Frequent Meals: Aim for six smaller meals each day rather than three substantial ones. This method makes it easier to prevent overfeeding the stomach and facilitates faster emptying.

2. Chew deeply: Chewing food deeply can help alleviate symptoms and facilitate digestion. Make sure that the food is broken down into smaller, more digestible bits by taking your time with each bite.

3. Sit Upright After Eating: After eating, stay seated for a minimum of one to two hours. By using gravity, this aids in the passage of food through the digestive system.

4. Avoid Eating Before Bedtime: To avoid symptoms at night and to give your stomach enough time to empty before lying down, try not to eat within three hours of going to bed.

Choices and Food Preparation

Food preparation methods and selections have a big influence on how symptoms are managed:

1. Cooked vs. Raw: Since cooking breaks down fiber and facilitates digestion, choose cooked foods over raw ones. Soups, stews, and soft-cooked veggies provide great options.

2. Smoothies and Purees: Foods can be easier to digest and yet contain vital nutrients when blended into smoothies or purees. This is very beneficial for veggies and fruits.

3. Low-Fiber Foods: To prevent aggravating symptoms, select low-fiber foods. Although soluble fiber from foods like oatmeal and peeled fruits is often better tolerated than insoluble fiber, soluble fiber is still needed.

4. Intake of Fat: To avoid delaying stomach emptying, cut back on foods high in fat. Moderately choose fats that are better for you, including those in avocados and olive oil.

Hydration

For everyone, but especially for those who have gastroparesis, staying hydrated is essential. The following advice can help you stay well hydrated:

1. Drink Fluids Throughout the Day: Spread out your fluid intake throughout the day rather than consuming huge amounts at once. By doing this, pain and sensations of fullness may be avoided.

2. Electrolyte Solutions: If you feel like you're throwing up, think about taking electrolyte solutions or sports drinks. These can support hydration and the replacement of lost nutrients.

3. Avoid Carbonated Beverages: These beverages can make you feel uncomfortable and bloated. Remain with non-carbonated drinks such as clear broths, herbal teas, and water.

Exercise

Frequent exercise can help with digestion and enhance general health. But it's crucial to adjust activities to each person's strengths and weaknesses:

1. Light Exercise: To aid in promoting digestion, stroll or do little exercise after meals. Even a quick stroll might have a big impact.

2. Gentle Yoga: Yoga is beneficial, especially the poses that stretch and twist the abdomen gently. Additionally, yoga helps people unwind and reduce tension.

3. Avoid Strenuous Activity: Excessive exercise just after a meal may have the opposite effect. Give yourself at least an hour to recover from a meal before doing more strenuous exercise.

Stress Reduction

Anxiety and stress can make gastroparesis symptoms worse. Including stress-reduction methods in your everyday activities can be beneficial.

Mindfulness and Meditation : Techniques like these can help people feel less stressed and more at ease. Deep breathing techniques can be helpful even for a short while.

2. Support Groups: By joining a support group, people with gastroparesis can get both practical and emotional assistance from like-minded individuals.

3. Counseling: To help manage anxiety and despair that may result from having a chronic illness, think about seeking professional counseling or therapy.

Handling Medication

In order to reduce problems and control symptoms of gastroparesis, proper pharmaceutical management is essential:

1. Follow Prescriptions: Make sure you take your prescriptions exactly as directed by your doctor. Never change a dosage without first talking to your doctor.

2. Medication Timing: Certain medications may need to be taken in accordance with meal schedules. Make sure you comprehend and adhere to the directions.

3. Report adverse Effects: Notify your healthcare practitioner of any pharmaceutical adverse effects you may be experiencing. They might have to modify your treatment regimen.

Frequent Medical Check-Ups

Scheduling routine check-ups with your physician is crucial for keeping an eye on and treating gastroparesis:

1. Regular Check-ups: By tracking your condition and making the required modifications to your treatment plan, routine check-ups can help.

2. Nutritional evaluations: A dietitian can conduct periodic evaluations to make sure you are getting enough nutrition and to make any dietary changes that may be required.

3. Observe Symptoms: Maintain a symptom journal to record the meals and activities that set off symptoms. To help customize your treatment strategy, supply your healthcare professional with this information.

Emotional and Social Welfare

Having gastroparesis can have an impact on your emotional and social life. It is imperative to attend to these facets:

1. Remain Socially Connected: Keep up relationships with loved ones and friends. Try to maintain social engagement as isolation can deteriorate emotional health.

2. Plan Ahead: When you go to social gatherings, make sure you bring safe foods or let the host know about any dietary restrictions you may have.

3. Seek Support: To assist you deal with the emotional difficulties of having a chronic illness, don't be afraid to ask for help from close friends and family or from qualified counselors.

126

Modifying Through Time

Since gastroparesis is a disorder that might alter over time, it's critical to manage it with flexibility and adaptability:

1. Remain Up to Date: Stay informed on the most recent findings and research regarding gastroparesis. There may be dietary changes and new medical procedures that can enhance your quality of life.

2. Adjust as Needed: Be ready to modify your treatment strategy, food, and way of life in response to changes in your tolerance and symptoms.

3. Preserve Hope: Although gastroparesis might be difficult to live with, it is possible to control symptoms and have a happy life with the correct techniques and assistance.

A comprehensive strategy involving dietary modifications, lifestyle alterations, and routine medical treatment is required to manage gastroparesis. Seniors can improve their general quality of life, better manage their symptoms, and improve their nutritional condition by implementing these lifestyle guidelines. Recall that each person's experience with gastroparesis is unique, and it will take patience and time to find the proper balance of strategies. Despite the difficulties associated with gastroparesis, it is possible to live a pleasant and meaningful life with persistence and assistance.

127

Conclusion

There are particular difficulties associated with having gastroparesis, particularly for elderly people who may already be managing other medical issues and the aging process. But as this book has shown, it is feasible to effectively manage gastroparesis with careful food selections, lifestyle modifications, and proactive healthcare management. Although each person's experience with gastroparesis is unique and highly personal, it is possible to lead a happy and healthy life if you have the correct information and resources.

Contemplating Nutritional Control

A properly planned diet that strikes a balance between nourishment and the need to reduce symptoms is the cornerstone of controlling gastroparesis. The Gastroparesis Diet Cookbook for Seniors offers a selection of foods that are meant to be easy on the stomach while yet providing vital nutrients. It is impossible to overestimate the significance of modest, frequent meals. Large meals should be avoided in favor of foods that are quick to digest, as this will aid in faster stomach emptying, less discomfort, and improved digestion in general.

This cookbook's recipes are designed with seniors with gastroparesis in mind. Every meal, from hearty breakfast selections like oatmeal and soft scrambled eggs to filling lunch and dinner ideas like pureed vegetable soups and delicate baked salmon, is thoughtfully prepared. You will have plenty of options to sustain your energy levels and stay hydrated throughout the day thanks to the snacks and beverages that are included. You may construct a fun and interesting diet that promotes your health by experimenting with these recipes and modifying them to suit your individual tastes and dietary requirements.

Value of Tailored Dietary Practices

The value of customized nutrition is one of the main points this book makes. Every person with gastroparesis is affected differently, so what works for one may not work for another. Maintaining a food journal can be a very useful tool for figuring out what foods cause symptoms and which ones are well tolerated. This enables you to modify your meal plans in accordance with your informed dietary decisions.

Additional support can be obtained by working with a dietician or nutritionist who is knowledgeable about gastroparesis. These experts can guide you through dietary limitations, make sure you're getting enough nutrition, and provide helpful guidance on meal preparation and planning. In order to cover any nutritional deficiencies, they can also assist you in incorporating essential dietary supplements. These supplements, which are frequently required because of restricted food intake, include multivitamins, calcium, vitamin D, and iron.

When it comes to controlling gastroparesis, diet is simply one factor in the equation. Changes in lifestyle are essential for managing symptoms and promoting general wellbeing. Small adjustments can have a big impact on how well your digestive system processes food. Some examples of these adjustments include eating smaller, more frequent meals, chewing food well, and remaining upright after eating.

Exercise is also another crucial component. Walking is a simple form of gentle exercise that can assist improve general health and increase digestion. Relaxation and stress reduction can also be facilitated by gentle yoga and other low-impact exercises. Finding the right balance between staying active enough to maintain your digestive health and avoiding physically demanding activities right after eating is crucial.

Since stress can make symptoms of gastroparesis worse, stress management is essential. Deep breathing exercises, meditation, and mindfulness are some of the techniques that might help you stay calm and manage stress. You can get emotional support and learn coping mechanisms for managing the difficulties of having a chronic illness by attending support groups or getting counseling.

The Function of Medical Administration

Having routine medical check-ups is crucial to effectively manage gastroparesis. Regular check-ups with your healthcare practitioner enable continuous condition monitoring and necessary modifications to your treatment plan. This can involve managing prescription drugs, evaluating diets, and taking care of any other potential health problems.

Prokinetics and antiemetics are two examples of gastroparesis medications that can help control symptoms by encouraging stomach emptying and lowering nausea and vomiting. It's critical that you take these drugs as directed and let your doctor know if you have any adverse effects. If symptoms are severe and not effectively controlled with existing therapies, surgery may be considered in certain circumstances.

Social and Emotional Welfare

Having gastroparesis can have an adverse effect on your social and emotional health. It's critical to address these issues and figure out how to continue living a happy and fulfilled life. Finding ways to engage in social interactions and activities without sacrificing your nutritional needs is essential for mental well-being. You can stay involved with family and friends by bringing your own safe foods, stating your dietary restrictions to hosts, and making advance plans for social activities.

Support groups, therapists, and other family members can offer emotional support that fosters a sense of belonging and mutual understanding. It can bring great comfort and empowerment to know that you are not traveling alone. In order to achieve total well-being, it is critical to treat any emotions of worry, despair, or isolation. Mental health is equally as vital as physical health.

Adjusting and Maintaining Knowledge

Since gastroparesis is a condition that might alter over time, it's critical to maintain an adaptable and flexible approach to care. Making educated decisions about your health can be facilitated by keeping up with the most recent findings and available treatments. There might be updates to food guidelines, drug recommendations, and therapy interventions that provide new symptom management options.

Being proactive with your health entails keeping your doctor and yourself informed on a regular basis, keeping an eye out for any signs, and being prepared to modify your lifestyle and nutrition as necessary. It's critical to have hope and a positive attitude because, although managing a chronic illness can be difficult, it is still possible to have a happy, fulfilled life with the correct support and techniques.

Looking Ahead

Recall that managing gastroparesis is a dynamic and continuous activity as you proceed on your path with it. This cookbook's techniques and recipes are meant to provide you with a solid basis for handling your symptoms and preserving your health. You can safely treat gastroparesis and enhance your quality of life by combining food control, lifestyle changes, and routine medical care.

Accept the help of your family, friends, and medical team, and don't be afraid to look for new sources of knowledge and resources. Every action you take to improve your gastroparesis management is one step closer to living a longer, healthier life. Remain knowledgeable, patient, and—above all—hopeful. There may be ups and downs in your gastroparesis path, but with the correct strategy, you may overcome these obstacles and prosper.

In summary, managing gastroparesis involves a multimodal strategy that includes medication, lifestyle, food, and mental health. You now have the information and resources necessary to effectively manage your illness and make well-informed decisions about your health thanks to this book. Recall that there are numerous tools and support networks at your disposal to assist you on your journey, and you are not alone. Despite the difficulties caused by gastroparesis, you can have a healthy and satisfying life by adopting a proactive and optimistic outlook. We are grateful that you have included our cookbook in your quest for improved health and wellbeing.

www.ingramcontent.com/pod-product-compliance
Lightning Source LLC
Chambersburg PA
CBHW071930210526
45479CB00002B/621